The 20 Week Osbon Total Body Transformation

and
Bonus workout plan

By David Huskey

Congratulations you are about to embark on the hardest and most rewarding 20 weeks of your life. No matter how hard it gets stick with this program for the full 20 weeks it will be a life changing process that will leave you completely transformed at the end. Take before pictures and pictures after completing each section to keep you motivated your friends and family will notice huge changes within a short period of time. Again congratulations on taking this important step towards your health and wellbeing. Let's get started

Week 1-3

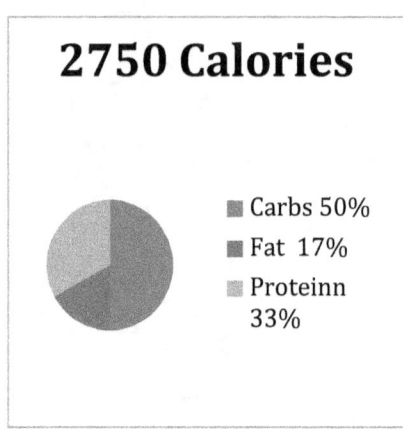

2750 Calories

- Carbs 50%
- Fat 17%
- Proteinn 33%

Week 1 through 3 will be upping your calorie intake and limiting the calories from each of the three groups in the graph.

345 Grams of Carbs
225 Grams of Protein
50 Grams of Fat

Plan out your meals the night before you can eat whatever you want just make sure to stay under the weekly carb, protein, and fat levels.

It is easier if plan out breakfast, lunch, and dinner with snacks in between the meals a couple of days in advance at the very least the night before. Do not go over the amounts allowed if a food puts you over change it. This is critical in fixing your body's metabolism. We need to retrain your body into processing foods correctly.

Week 4-7

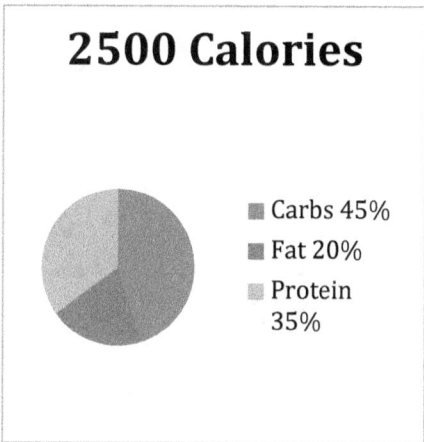

2500 Calories

- ■ Carbs 45%
- ■ Fat 20%
- ■ Protein 35%

Week 4-7 Calorie intake drops to 2500 calories and you need to adjust the carbs, fat, and protein to hit the correct percentage.

281 grams of carbs
218 grams of protein
55   grams of Fat

Again it is extremely important to follow these ratios and to pre plan your meals so you know exactly what you can eat without going over the numbers do not try and do it on the fly you will mess up and go over the numbers. I know it's difficult but stay with it!

week 8-12

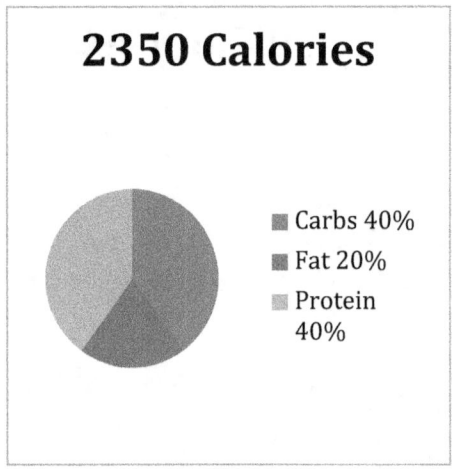

2350 Calories

- Carbs 40%
- Fat 20%
- Protein 40%

Ok week 8-12 is going to be a lot easier you are almost there by now you have noticed some huge changes stick with the goals for this section and finish out strong.

Again the calorie intake has changed and also the percentage of each area intake has changed keep up with the meal planning and stick to these requirements.

235 grams of carbs
235 grams of Protein
52 grams of Fat

Week 13-16

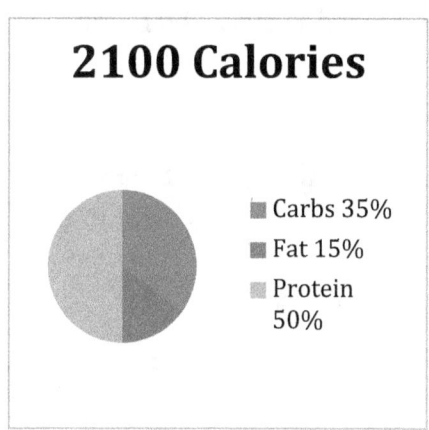

2100 Calories

- Carbs 35%
- Fat 15%
- Protein 50%

Week 13-16 we are going to start adjusting the protein, carbs , and fat intakes pretty significantly this will take a lot more meal planning to ensure you hit the calorie intake without going over the requirements.

183 grams of carbs
262 grams of protein
35   grams of Fat

Congratulations on making it this far you are almost there keep going and don't give up!

Week 17-20

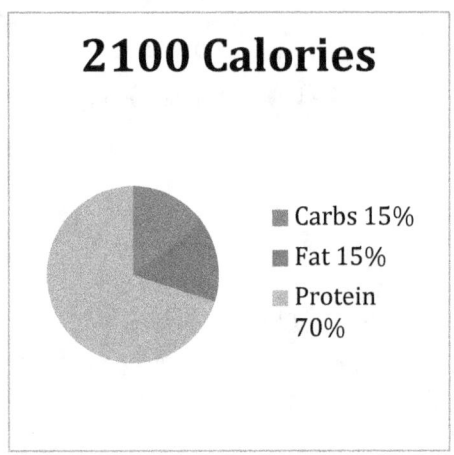

2100 Calories

- Carbs 15%
- Fat 15%
- Protein 70%

Week 17-20 this is the final section and one of the hardest to keep on target so stay with it and get ready to celebrate you have earned it.

78 grams of Carbs
367 grams of Protein
35 grams of Fat

Congratulations you have completed the 20 week Osbon total body transformation as a gift to you for all of your hard work and dedication is a bonus work out plan.

Thank you for your purchase and following my diet and workout plan. I hope the results have been as life changing for you as they have been for so many others. Congratulations again and remember to share this program with family, friends, or anyone that could benefit from a total body transformation.

Bonus Workout plan

Main Focus:
Shoulders
Upper Chest
Arms
Back

Chest/Shoulders/Biceps

Flat Barbell Bench
4 Sets of 8-12reps
These should be HEAVY. I want GOOD reps. It should be hard to get to 8-12
In between each set you will perform a triple super set of Front, Lateral, and Rear Delt Raises – 12reps

Incline Smith Machine or Incline Bench Press
4 Sets of 8-12reps
These should HEAVY. I want GOOD reps. It should be hard to get to 8-12
In between each set you will perform a super set of Lateral Raises and Rear Delt Raises – 12Reps

Incline Dumbbell Bench/Barbell Curls as a SuperSet
4 Sets of 8-12reps
These should HEAVY. I want GOOD reps. It should be hard to get to 8-12
After each set of Bench – Barbell Curls 4 Sets of 8-12Reps

Incline Flys/DB Hammer Curls
4 Sets of 8-12Reps
After each set of Incline Flys – SuperSet with DB Hammer Curls
4 Sets of 8-12Reps

Cable Flys/Dips for Chest
This is a super set
For the Cable Flys – Lightweight – Good stretch with a good squeeze
4 sets of 12 reps
For the Dips
All the way up, all the way down with a squeeze at the top. Reps are to failure, but make the reps perfect

Arms

Pullups
4 Sets to Failure

One Arm Reverse Tricep Extensions
4 Sets of 8-12reps
These should be HEAVY. I want GOOD reps. It should be hard to get to 8-12

Straight Bar Curls
4 Sets of 8-12reps
These should be HEAVY. I want GOOD reps. It should be hard to get to 8-12

Dumbbell Overhead Tricep Press
4 Sets of 8-12reps
These should be HEAVY. I want GOOD reps. It should be hard to get to 8-12

Dumbbell Preacher Curls
4 Sets of 8-12reps
These should be HEAVY. I want GOOD reps. It should be hard to get to 8-12

VBar or EZ Bar Cable Tricep Press Downs
4 Sets of 8-12reps
These should be HEAVY. I want GOOD reps. It should be hard to get to 8-12

Hammer Curls
4 Sets of 8-12reps
These should be HEAVY. I want GOOD reps. It should be hard to get to 8-12

Triceps Kickbacks
7 Sets of 10-12Reps
Good Reps – Oh and you only get 1min for Rest

DB Inside Curls
7 Sets of 10-12Reps
Good Reps – 1min for Rest
These are to be done with the same motion you would use if you were doing inside grip EZ Bar curls. But this is with DB.

Legs

Squats
4 Sets of 8-12reps
These should be HEAVY. I want GOOD reps. It should be hard to
get to 8-12

Leg Press
4 Sets of 8-12reps
These should be HEAVY. I want GOOD reps. It should be hard to
get to 8-12

Barbell Lunges
4 Sets of 8-12reps
These should be HEAVY. I want GOOD reps. It should be hard to
get to 8-12

Leg Extensions
4 Sets of 12-14reps
Pay attention to the squeeze at the top – Do not bounce

Leg Curls
4 Sets of 8-12reps
These should be HEAVY. I want GOOD reps. It should be hard to
get to 8-12

Standing Calf Raises
4 Sets of 8-12 Perfect Reps – Then go until failure

Seated Calf Raises
4 Sets of 8-12 Perfect Reps – Then go until failure

Shoulders/Triceps

Smith Machine Shoulder Press
4 Sets of 8-12reps
These should be HEAVY. I want GOOD reps. It should be hard to
get to 8-12

DB Shoulder Press
Dumbbell Shoulder Press
4 Sets of 8-12reps
These should be HEAVY. I want GOOD reps. It should be hard to
get to 8-12

Front Raises
4 Sets of 8-12reps
These should be HEAVY. I want GOOD reps. It should be hard to
get to 8-12

Lateral Raises
4 Sets of 8-12reps
These should be HEAVY. I want GOOD reps. It should be hard to
get to 8-12

Rear Raises
4 Sets of 8-12reps

These should be HEAVY. I want GOOD reps. It should be hard to get to 8-12

Barbell Shrugs
4 Sets of 8-12reps
These should be HEAVY. I want GOOD reps. It should be hard to get to 8-12

7 Sets of 10 – 1min Rest
Front or Lateral or Rear Dumbbell Raises – Pick one and alternate each week
All I'm looking for is for you to exhaust the muscle completely.

Single Arm Reverse Cable Tri Extension
4 Sets of 8-12reps
These should be HEAVY. I want GOOD reps. It should be hard to get to 8-12

EZ Bar or VBar Tricep Extensions
4 Sets of 8-12reps
These should be HEAVY. I want GOOD reps. It should be hard to get to 8-12

Back
With all of your back workouts, really concentrate on squeezing at the end of the movement. Do not bounce.

Deadlifts
4 Sets of 8-12reps
These should be HEAVY. I want GOOD reps. It should be hard to get to 8-12

Pullups – Weighted if you can

4 Sets – Good Reps, with wide grip as you can go. Try for 10Reps for each set minimum
Between Each Set – Front and Lateral Raises for Shoulders
4 Sets of 10-12Reps

Lat Pulldowns
4 Sets of 8-12reps
These should be HEAVY. I want GOOD reps. It should be hard to get to 8-12

Bent Over Row
4 Sets of 8-12reps
These should be HEAVY. I want GOOD reps. It should be hard to get to 8-12
Make sure to squeeze at the top – NO BOUNCING

Middle Grip – NOT CLOSED GRIP – Lat Pulldown
4 Sets of 8-12reps
These should be HEAVY. I want GOOD reps. It should be hard to get to 8-12

Seated Cable Rows
4 Sets of 8-12reps
These should be HEAVY. I want GOOD reps. It should be hard to get to 8-12

Straight Arm Cable Pulldowns for Lats
7 Stes of 10Reps with 20 second rest in between

Congratulations

I hope you completed both the 20 week Osbon total body transformation and the accompanied workout plan.

A lot of planning and effort went into creating this program. I hope it brings as much success to your life as it has to mine.

I was struggling with diabetes and was at 240 pounds after a lot of trial and error and talking to many specialists and a lot of collaboration the 20 week Osbon total body transformation was created. I now am at a consistent 172 pounds and no longer require Insulin. This program truly is a life changing experience. It is not an easy process as I am sure you have found out over the 20 weeks. If you didn't complete the whole program and slipped up and stopped altogether go back and try again. You will be better prepared for the rigors of the program. Now that you know what to expect create a meal plan for the entire 20 week program so you know what to do each day.

Total body transformation

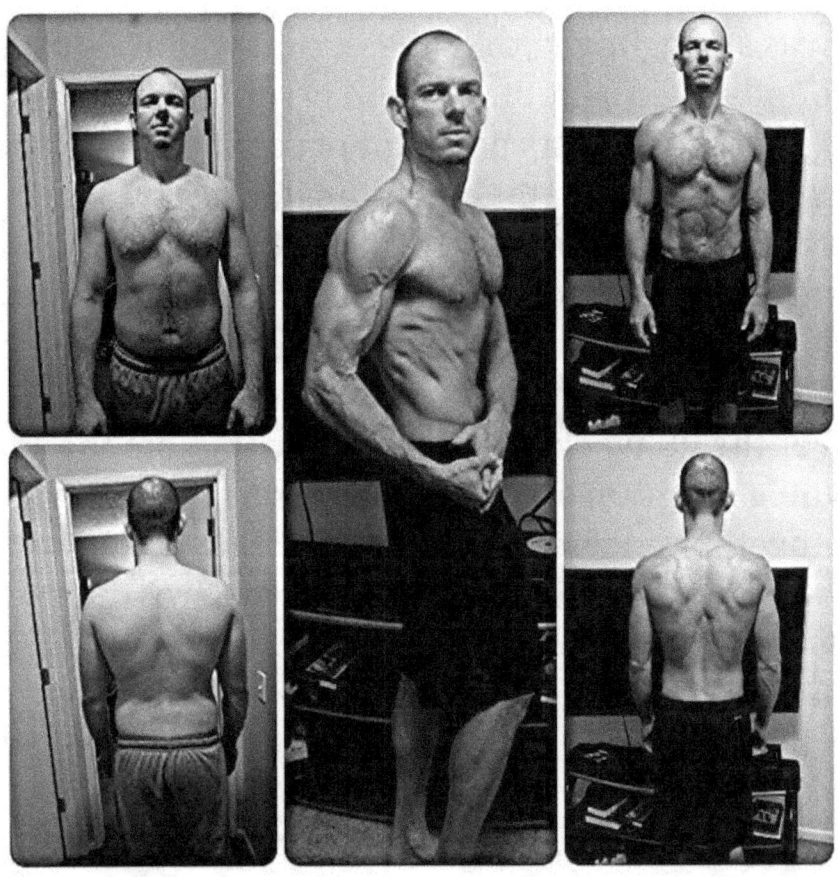

Week 1-3

Starting weight –

Starting picture   After week 3
picture

Week 4-7

weight –

Starting picture
picture

After week 7

Week 8-12

weight –

Starting picture
picture

After week 12

Week 13-16

 weight –

Starting picture   After week 16
picture

Week 17-20

weight –

Starting picture
picture

After week 20

Notes